A Complete Overview of Breast Health

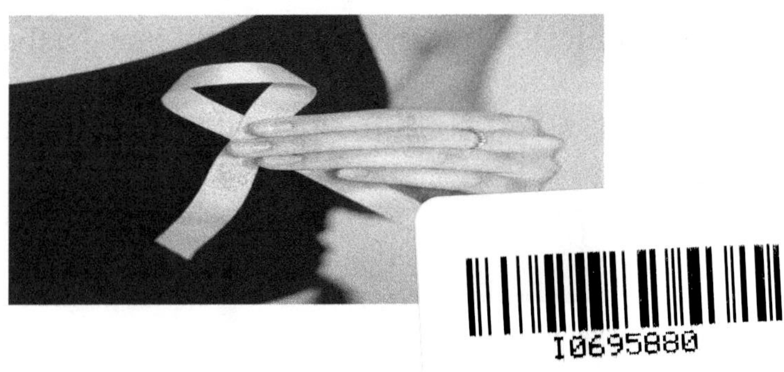

Angel B. Maurice

Table of Contents

INTRODUCTION

The mission of Breast Cancer Awareness is to Shine a Light on Hope and Empower Lives.

When it comes to the fabric of human health, there are very few obstacles that reverberate as powerfully as the never-ending fight against breast cancer. This introduction acts as a compass to guide us through the complex terrain of breast cancer awareness, which is a communal endeavor to shed light on the possibility of a cure and to empower individuals' lives. As we get started on this trip, we delve into the heart of this prevalent health condition. We do this because we recognize how important it is to raise awareness about an illness that affects the lives of millions of people all over the world.

Cancer of the breast is a fierce foe that has no demographic borders; it strikes women and, in extremely rare cases, males of any age, race, or socioeconomic level; it does not discriminate. Because of the complexity of its makeup, not only does it require medical comprehension, but also wider societal recognition. In the following chapters, we will attempt to decipher the complexities of breast cancer by providing insights into its roots, the factors that contribute to its prevalence, and the diverse manifestations that it can take.

Our inquiry starts with a general introduction to breast cancer, during which we will strip away the layers to discover the complexities of this disease. From there, we go on to the significance of awareness, which serves as a compass pointing individuals and communities in the same direction so that they can stand together in their quest for information, early detection, and ultimately, victory against adversity.

To fully comprehend breast cancer, one needs to take a sophisticated approach. In the following sections, we will examine the causes and risk factors that contributed to its development. Our discussion focuses on the numerous subtypes of breast cancer, each of which has a unique set of symptoms and necessitates a specialized approach to diagnosis and treatment. The indications and symptoms that serve as early whispers, motivating proactive involvement with one's health, are discussed in detail throughout these pages for the reader's perusal.

The emphasis placed on early detection and screening is one of the most important aspects of the awareness theme. As the chapters go, they provide instructions on how to perform breast self-exams, discuss the relevance of clinical breast exams, and outline the function that mammograms play in detecting potential risks before they become more severe. Knowledge is a potent ally in the fight against breast cancer, and the only way for individuals to take care of their own health and well-being is to make decisions that are based on accurate information.

The story then smoothly transitions into the various therapeutic possibilities that are open to the patient. Unveiling surgical interventions, chemotherapy, radiation therapy, targeted therapy, hormone therapy, and immunotherapy, as well as providing a comprehensive understanding of the various strategies utilized in the fight against breast cancer, are the goals of this article. Real-life accounts of survivors woven throughout the text shed light on the tenacity and fortitude inherent in the human spirit, thereby igniting a desire for hope and a resolve to overcome obstacles.

As we progress along our individual paths to success, the significance of having support systems becomes increasingly apparent. The roles that families and friends play are discussed, and it is acknowledged that the emotional support that these relationships offer is an essential component of the recovery process.

Within the context of our collective response to breast cancer, prevention appears as an essential component. Modifications to one's way of life, genetic counseling, and testing are broken down in this book, providing readers with actionable insights into reducing exposure to potential health hazards and taking charge of their own health care.

This investigation goes beyond the scope of individual conflicts. We delve into international initiatives as well as grassroots movements, and we celebrate the progress that has been made in advocacy and awareness campaigns. The focus here is on organizations that are tirelessly working to elevate the conversation surrounding breast cancer, thereby helping to foster a sense of community and a shared sense of purpose.

In the concluding chapters, we highlight important resources and support organizations as a means of throwing a lifeline to readers who are looking for direction and assistance. The conclusion acts as a rallying cry, inviting readers to contribute to the ongoing fight against breast cancer. This helps to ensure that the light of awareness continues to shine brightly.

In this beautiful symphony of understanding and compassion, our combined efforts resound with the message that raising awareness about breast cancer is more than just a campaign; it is a movement, a driving force that changes lives and shapes a future in which hope prevails over adversity. Join us as we navigate this complex tapestry, weaving together understanding, resilience, and the unwavering belief that, together, we can prevail over whatever challenges we face.

CHAPTER 1

Unraveling the Complicated Nature of
Breast Cancer and Its Understanding

One of the most important cornerstones in the complex landscape that is healthcare is having a solid understanding of breast cancer. We must pay attention, show empathy, and make a concerted effort to better understand the intricacies of breast cancer because this adversary is multifaceted and frequently inscrutable. This chapter acts as a guide by removing the layers to uncover the complexities of this ubiquitous sickness. It investigates the roots of the disease, the elements that lead to its emergence, and the various symptoms that it can take.

The term "breast cancer" actually refers to a diverse group of diseases that all have one thing in common: they all affect the breast tissues. Breast cancer is not a single disease. Before we can begin to understand the complexities of it, we must first recognize the many forms it can take. Each subtype of breast cancer, from ductal carcinoma in situ to invasive lobular carcinoma, offers its own distinct set of difficulties, which calls for individualized approaches to diagnosis, treatment, and survivorship. By gaining an understanding of these disparities, individuals can gain the power of knowledge, which enables them to make educated decisions and fosters a proactive attitude toward health.

There is likely more than one thing that led to the development of breast cancer, both in terms of causation and risk factors. This condition is caused by a complicated interaction between predispositions that are passed down through generations, hormonal factors, and the decisions that people make about how they live their lives. This chapter goes into the maze of causes, illuminating the intricate web of effects that may either exacerbate or lessen the risk. By unraveling these threads, we provide individuals the ability to evaluate and alter their risk profiles, offering a path toward prevention in the process.

As we move through the chapters, the signs and symptoms that the body employs to communicate possible dangers take center stage. These signals and symptoms constitute a silent language. From minor changes in breast texture to the detection of a lump, knowing these indicators becomes paramount. Knowledge converts into a tool for early detection, a cornerstone in the broader strategy of controlling breast cancer effectively.

The road to understanding breast cancer is not only clinical; it is extremely human. Real tales of individuals who have faced this illness head-on weave through the narrative, revealing glimpses into the fortitude, perseverance, and hope that characterize the breast cancer journey. These accounts serve as beacons, illuminating the route for individuals navigating their own struggles and bringing solace to those in search of common experiences.

Central to our investigation is the awareness that breast cancer is not an isolated problem but a common experience that resonates globally. This chapter unfolds the narrative of breast cancer on a greater scale, reflecting its influence across many communities, cultures, and societies. It urges readers to engage with the worldwide conversation on breast cancer, developing empathy, understanding, and collaborative efforts to confront this difficult health crisis.

As we explore the complexity of breast cancer, this chapter stands as a monument to the importance of information in navigating the complications of healthcare. Understanding breast cancer transcends medical textbooks; it demands a comprehensive vision that covers the person, the community, and the global collective. It is through this complex understanding that we may construct a path toward prevention, early detection, and, ultimately, triumph over breast cancer's strong presence. Join us on this journey of comprehension and empathy as we endeavor to unravel the nuances of breast cancer, one revelation at a time.

CHAPTER 2

Early Detection and Screening: Illuminating Paths to Timely Intervention

In the world of breast cancer, early diagnosis emerges as a strong ally, a beacon that illuminates routes to prompt intervention and improved outcomes. This chapter is devoted to elucidating the complexities of early detection and screening, with the overarching goal of highlighting the central role that these aspects play in the overall strategy against breast cancer. Each stage, from the personal nature of breast self-examinations to the objective nature of clinical screens and mammograms, contributes to the overarching mission of recognizing potential dangers in their earliest stages so that appropriate preventative measures can be taken.

The story starts off with an investigation into breast self-exams, which are described as an "intimate journey" in which "individuals become the primary architects of their health." One can develop a sensitivity to the minute shifts that occur in breast tissue using palpation and observation, and this makes it possible to identify abnormalities in their earliest stages. This chapter is intended to serve as a guide, offering insights into the methodology, frequency, and significance of self-examinations, with an emphasis on the power that resides in knowing one's own body.

Clinical breast exams are an important link in the chain of early detection. These exams are performed by medical experts and take place in a clinical setting. This section digs deeper into the methodical technique of clinical examinations, in which experienced medical professionals navigate the terrain of breast tissue to find probable abnormalities that might need additional research. Because of the collaborative nature of these examinations, it is essential for individuals to maintain frequent checkups with their healthcare professionals and have open lines of communication with those physicians.

In the following section, mammography, an essential part of breast cancer screening, will be given the spotlight it deserves. This imaging technology makes use of low-dose X-rays to acquire detailed images of breast tissue. As a result, it makes it possible to discover abnormalities in the breast tissue that could be missed by other methods. The chapter guides the reader through the complexities of mammography and addresses typical issues, such as when to begin screenings and how to interpret the importance of the findings. It highlights the significance of mammography as an effective weapon in the fight against breast cancer, which significantly increases the likelihood of early identification and prompt treatment.

The process of gaining an understanding of the landscape of early detection is not limited to the efforts of individuals alone; rather, it encompasses the endeavors of an entire community as well as healthcare regulations. This chapter examines the significance of having easy access to screening programs, the part that awareness campaigns play in encouraging people to take part in screenings, and the continuous research that is aimed at enhancing and broadening screening procedures. It recognizes that early detection is a collaborative effort that calls for the dedication and assistance of the society as a whole.

There are personal accounts of people whose lives have been changed as a result of the application of early detection interspersed throughout the tale. These first-person tales shed light on the significant impact that prompt intervention can have, highlighting the potentially game-changing role that screenings can play in creating the kinds of outcomes that are favorable. These tales act as guiding lights, encouraging individuals to participate in routine screenings and communities to make investments in complete healthcare infrastructure.

This chapter encourages readers to regard early diagnosis and screening not as isolated events but rather as integral components of a larger strategy against breast cancer. As we negotiate the terrain of early detection and screening, we invite readers to view these practices not as isolated events but rather as integrated components. It is a call to action, urging individuals, communities, and healthcare systems to collaborate in the pursuit of early detection, an endeavor that holds the promise of transforming the trajectory of breast cancer from a formidable challenge into a triumph of resilience and proactivity. It reinforces the notion that awareness is not a passive concept; rather, it is a call to action.

CHAPTER 3

Treatment Alternatives: How to Make Your Way Through the Maze of Breast Cancer Care

Treatment options emerge as crucial threads within the complex tapestry that is breast cancer, stitching together a story of perseverance and hope in the process. This chapter delves into the various tactics that are being used in the fight against breast cancer, a battle in which technological advances in medicine and individualized treatment are converging to meet the specific requirements of every person who is up against this strong foe.

Surgery, which is frequently the first step in the fight against breast cancer, takes the spotlight in this part of our investigation. In this part, the complexities of various surgical procedures, ranging from lumpectomies, which leave some of the breast tissue intact, to mastectomies, which, when necessary, remove the entire breast, are untangled. The surgical options are presented not only as processes, but also as individualized choices that are directed by the particulars of each condition. This gives patients the ability to make educated judgments about the courses of treatment they will follow.

The use of chemotherapy, a tried-and-true weapon in the fight against cancer, will be the focus of the next stage of our investigation. This comprehensive treatment makes use of potent medications to specifically target and eradicate cancer cells located anywhere in the body. The reader is taken on a journey through the terrain of chemotherapy, during which they get insights into its mechanics, probable side effects, and the developing field of tailored therapies, which attempt to boost efficacy while minimizing unpleasant responses. This chapter highlights the collaborative nature of cancer care, which requires both patients and healthcare practitioners to work together to manage the obstacles and triumphs of therapy.

In the following paragraphs, we will examine radiation therapy, which is a method of treating cancer that is both targeted and highly specific. This therapy targets cancer cells by utilizing high doses of radiation, and it can be administered either after surgery to eliminate any leftover cancer cells or as a stand-alone treatment. The story delves into the intricacies of radiation therapy, illuminating its function as a means of preventing the loss of breast tissue and elevating the overall success rates of treatment.

The landscape of breast cancer care extends beyond conventional treatments and delves into targeted therapy, which is a field of precision medicine that zeroes in on specific molecular properties of cancer cells. This shift in the landscape of breast cancer care has implications for the future of cancer care. This part guides the listener through the ever-changing landscape of targeted interventions, including HER2-targeted medications and hormone therapy that address hormone receptor-positive breast tumors. It also provides a glimpse into the potential of personalized cancer care in the future.

The final component of our investigation is immunotherapy, which is a ground-breaking area in the treatment of cancer. Immunotherapy is a revolutionary new strategy for cancer treatment since it targets and eliminates cancer cells by utilizing the body's own immune system. In this section, the potential of immunotherapy in the context of breast cancer is unveiled, and a glimpse into ongoing research and the potentially life-changing impact it could have for patients coping with a breast cancer diagnosis is provided.

The stories of individuals who have overcome adversity and emerged on the other side with resilience and hope are interspersed throughout this chapter. These individuals have successfully navigated the maze of available treatment alternatives. These narratives lend a feeling of humanity to the professional debates by demonstrating that the goal of treatment is not merely the destruction of cancer cells but also the maintenance of a high quality of life and the development of a strong sense of agency in the face of adversity.

The readers will encounter a variety of therapy alternatives, but the overall theme is one of empowerment throughout their journey. Each decision that is provided is not a need but rather a possibility, and it is influenced by the people's interactions with their own healthcare teams. This chapter reaffirms the notion that breast cancer care is not an activity that can be simplified down to a single approach; rather, it is an evolving and individualized journey at the intersection of science and humanity that paves the way for individuals to negotiate the complexity of therapy with knowledge, fortitude, and a sense of hope.

CHAPTER 4

Survivor Stories: Celebrating Triumphs of Resilience in the Fight Against Breast Cancer

Amid the maze that is breast cancer, the experiences of those who have survived the disease emerge as moving testimonies to the unconquerable human spirit and the transformational power of perseverance. This chapter is an homage to people who have traversed the difficult terrain of diagnosis, treatment, and recovery. These are the individuals whose journeys reveal the road from vulnerability to strength, as well as the way from fear to hope.

The narratives of survivors form a mosaic, and inside that mosaic, diversity is king. Every person's experience is different, and together they create a tapestry that illustrates the complexities of living with breast cancer.

The reader embarks on a journey that goes beyond numbers and technical descriptions through these personal experiences, diving into the physical, emotional, and often victorious sides of survival.

The stories start at the moment when a diagnosis is made, which is the moment when people's lives are suddenly redirected into the unexplored area of uncertainty. These opening chapters are permeated by fear, perplexity, and a sense of vulnerability, representing the basic human response to the disclosure of a breast cancer diagnosis. Nevertheless, a germ of strength takes root within this common vulnerability, and it is nurtured by the inherent resilience that is present in individuals who face the unexpected with courage.

As the tales progress, it becomes clear that the therapy phase is a testing ground where both failure and success can be found. The reader is given a first-person account of the mental and physical toll that treatments such as surgery, chemotherapy, and radiation can take. These individual narratives demystify the clinical jargon by presenting treatment not as a sequence of medical operations but rather as a transforming journey that is distinguished by both moments of remarkable grace and times of intense struggle.

The narratives all share a common thread of lifelines in the form of recurring themes of support and connection. A person's family, friends, and healthcare providers become anchors during a storm because they provide encouragement, empathy, and a shared drive to triumph over the adversity. The significance of having a strong support network becomes more apparent, highlighting the team effort that is required throughout the breast cancer journey.

There are times of epiphany that occur during the challenges. These are profound realizations about the precarious nature of existence, the power that can be found in vulnerability, and the resiliency that is inherent in the human spirit. These times, which are frequently tucked away in the crevices of suffering and ambiguity, become guiding lights of optimism that shed light on the way forward for survivors and others who follow in their footsteps.

The post-treatment phase, which is characterized by periods of introspection and adjustment as well as a reevaluation of one's life priorities, is also discussed in this chapter. These accounts illustrate the resiliency that is necessary to negotiate the unfamiliar territory that is life after cancer and show that survival is not the end of the trip but rather a new beginning. As survivors learn to turn their experiences into forces for positive change, this phase is frequently characterized by recurring themes like as gratitude, a newfound sense of purpose, and a commitment to activism.

These accounts all accept that the path of every survivor is a work in progress; it is a constant evolution of the self that is shaped by the past but is not defined by it. This acknowledgment is woven throughout the stories. The individuals who are willing to share their experiences extend an invitation to the readers to be witnesses to their weaknesses, their victories, and the rewoven fabric of their lives.

The experiences of those who have survived terrible ordeals are more than just accounts of the past; they are living testimony to the resiliency of the human spirit. The reader is encouraged to bear witness to the beauty that emerges from hardship, the strength that is born of vulnerability, and the enduring legacy of hope that permeates the experience of being a survivor as they make their way through these chapters.

CHAPTER 5

How to Help Loved Ones Through the
Emotional Maze of Breast Cancer
Supporting loved ones who have breast
cancer

The role of supportive loved ones becomes an essential and sensitive presence within the delicate dance of breast cancer. This chapter carefully explores the emotional landscape that surrounds a breast cancer diagnosis, highlighting the important role that family and friends play in providing peace, understanding, and steadfast support during this difficult time. This narrative sheds light on the transformational power of empathy and connection at every stage of the experience, from the initial shock of receiving a diagnosis to the subtle challenges of treatment and recovery.

The journey starts with the moment of revelation, which is the discovery that you have breast cancer. Those who are close to the person who received the diagnosis often find themselves caught up in an emotional whirlwind as they attempt to balance their own anxieties and uncertainties with the need to be a source of support for the person who received the news. In this portion of the chapter, we examine the nuanced art of holding space, providing comfort, and sensitively navigating the early phases of the breast cancer journey.

The importance of the supportive roles played by family and friends becomes more apparent as the story progresses. The emotional ups and downs of treatment eventually become a shared experience that is characterized by both victories and setbacks. Family and friends are there to bear witness to the emotional and physical tolls that chemotherapy takes, as well as the day-to-day struggles that reframe what it means to be normal. This section provides some helpful insights on the difficult balance that must be struck while providing care for a person while at the same time ensuring that their agency and autonomy are not compromised.

It becomes clear that communication, which is essential to the success of any relationship, is the major theme. This chapter digs into the complexities of open communication and acknowledges the importance of words in the process of creating connection and comprehension. To create a space where vulnerability can be met with empathy and resilience, loved ones learn to navigate conversations that cross the range of emotions, from fear and despair to hope and joy. These conversations create a space for loved ones to learn how to talk to each other about their experiences.

To successfully navigate the emotional terrain requires more than just the ability to communicate verbally; it also incorporates the language of gestures, the art of performing acts of compassion, and the skill of just being present. This part examines the transformational power of simple, meaningful activities, such as making nourishing meals, offering an ear to listen, and creating joyful moments that punctuate the difficult road.

The emotional toll that can be taken by someone who provides care or support is acknowledged in this chapter as well. Those who care about us struggle with their own anxieties and feelings of powerlessness, even as they yearn to be rock-solid sources of support. Emerging themes of self-care and seeking help from supporters highlight the linked nature of an emotionally healthy path through breast cancer treatment.

As the story progresses, the time after therapy moves more and more into the spotlight. Those who care for breast cancer survivors negotiate the new territory of survivorship, celebrating victories but often coping with the complexities of life after the disease. This section provides some insights into the continuing significance of providing survivors and their loved ones with emotional assistance as they search for new ways to redefine and enhance their connections with one another.

Stories of overcoming adversity and testaments to the transformational power of love and support may be found interspersed throughout the chapter. These experiences reflect the essence of human connection, emphasizing that the breast cancer journey is not a solo path but rather a collective experience where shared vulnerability and shared strength intersect with one another.

To summarise, providing emotional support to loved ones who are coping with breast cancer is not a passive duty; rather, it is an active, ever-changing dance that requires empathy, communication, and consistent presence. This chapter encourages readers to acknowledge the transformative impact of their roles as supporters. It does so by pointing out that, in the symphony of feelings that surround breast cancer, the love and understanding provided by family and friends are notes that resonate profoundly, guiding individuals through the highs and lows of their transformative journey.

CHAPTER 6

Prevention of Breast Cancer: Reclaiming Control of Our Health and Our Lives through Proactive Health Strategies

In the vast terrain that is healthcare, the chapter on breast cancer prevention stands out like a beacon, revealing avenues to empower individuals in the proactive management of their own well-being. In the fight against breast cancer, prevention is a powerful ally that goes beyond simple awareness to include effective methods that modify lifestyles, encourage early diagnosis, and minimize risk factors. This article examines the myriad techniques of preventing breast cancer and emphasizes the fact that knowledge, when coupled with decisions made consciously, can be a transformative force in the pursuit of long-term physical well-being.

The investigation starts with a concentration on alterations in lifestyle, which are a fundamental component in the prevention of breast cancer. The maintenance of a healthy weight is dependent on a person's dietary practices, physical activity levels, and ability to stay active. This section digs deeper into the influence of nutrition and emphasizes the importance of eating a well-balanced diet that is high in fruits, vegetables, and whole grains. The story highlights the relevance of regular physical activity, highlighting how exercise not only contributes to overall health but also plays a role in reducing the risk of breast cancer. The narrative emphasizes the significance of regular physical activity and highlights how exercise contributes to overall health.

Genetic counseling and testing are an essential aspects of breast cancer prevention, in particular for people who come from medically affected families and have a history of the disease in their own lineage. Individuals gain the ability to make educated decisions regarding risk reduction after gaining a better understanding of the hereditary elements of breast cancer. This chapter delves into the complex realm of genetic counseling, shedding light on the repercussions of testing and the options that come after it.

The story eventually comes around to embracing the concept of breast self-awareness, which is a preventative measure that puts individuals in charge of their own healthcare decisions. Self-examination of the breasts regularly can serve as a technique for early detection by allowing individuals to recognize changes in their breast tissue and enabling them to seek immediate medical assistance when necessary. This section provides direction on the method of performing self-exams as well as the frequency of doing so, with an emphasis on the incorporation of self-awareness into regular health practices.

The significance of undergoing clinical screenings is brought to the forefront of the discussion as the chapter proceeds through topics such as routine breast checks and health checkups. Individuals and their healthcare providers must work together to achieve successful early identification of breast cancer, which is one of the most important aspects of breast cancer prevention. Individuals engage in a proactive posture against potential dangers when they submit themselves to routine screenings. This follows the notion that prevention is not only an individual responsibility but also a shared obligation within the context of the larger healthcare ecosystem.

The fight against breast cancer has expanded its scope to include the study of hormonal impacts and the maintenance of reproductive health. This part examines several factors, such as hormone replacement treatment and the timing of pregnancy and nursing, to shed light on the impact that these circumstances have in determining a woman's chance of developing breast cancer. When individuals are equipped with the information to understand these aspects, it becomes much easier for them to make informed decisions that are in line with their own personalized health goals.

The discussion comes to a close with a summary of the many approaches that have been discussed, with an emphasis on the fact that preventing breast cancer is an all-encompassing endeavor. Individuals can cultivate a culture of health that extends beyond their own actions to become the standard in society if they take the proactive step of adopting a proactive mindset and incorporating these tactics into their daily lives. This chapter reiterates the notion that the prevention of breast cancer is not merely a theoretical concept; rather, it is a real and practicable journey that individuals set out on daily, so molding their health destinies and contributing to a communal vision of a future in which breast cancer can not only be treated but also prevented.

Knowledge acts as the conductor in the symphony of breast cancer prevention, directing individuals to harmonize with practices that build health and resilience.

This chapter is an invitation—an invitation to adopt a proactive position, to prioritize well-being, and to recognize that each choice taken today is a step towards a future in which the incidence of breast cancer will have decreased and lives will be empowered through the transformational power of prevention.

CHAPTER 7

In the fight against breast cancer, advocacy, and awareness campaigns are helping to amplify the voices of those affected by the disease and spark change.

Campaigns become the megaphones that magnify voices, inspiring collective action and igniting change within the worldwide tapestry of breast cancer awareness. Advocacy develops as a driving force within the global tapestry of breast cancer awareness. This chapter serves as a monument to the dedicated efforts of advocates and the powerful initiatives that have impacted the conversation that surrounds breast cancer. The story develops, illuminating the transforming power of advocacy and the far-reaching influence of awareness campaigns. The story begins with local movements and moves on to multinational endeavors.

The first thing that this chapter does is establish what the essential function of advocacy is. Advocacy is defined as a dynamic force that goes beyond individual narratives to collectively impact policy, research, and public perception. Advocates are the builders of change, working persistently to de-stigmatize breast cancer, improve access to care, and foster an atmosphere where the global community is unified against this widespread health concern. Breast cancer is a common health challenge.

The grassroots movements that represent the spirit of local communities coming together in support of a common cause are the beating heart of the breast cancer awareness movement. This section investigates the beginnings of grass-roots movements and focuses on how ardent individuals, frequently those with a profoundly personal connection to breast cancer, have been the driving force behind grassroots movements that have had an effect on communities and fostered a sense of solidarity. The narrative demonstrates the capacity of everyday people to bring about exceptional change by looking at this phenomenon through the prism of grassroots advocacy.

As the narrative about breast cancer spreads to more countries throughout the world, the focus shifts to international organizations and campaigns. The investigation spans multiple continents and delves into endeavors that cut beyond national boundaries, cultural boundaries, and linguistic barriers. On a worldwide scale, these initiatives not only increase awareness but also affect legislation, having an impact on hospital infrastructure, research funding, and the general landscape of breast cancer care. This chapter takes a tour through historic campaigns that have made an unforgettable imprint on history, highlighting how public views and priorities can be reshaped via the use of strategic messaging and coordinated efforts.

The use of social media, which has emerged as a powerful instrument in the current period, is emerging as a game-changer in initiatives to raise awareness of breast cancer. Social media sites such as Twitter, Facebook, and Instagram have evolved into dynamic meeting places for activists to exchange personal narratives, communicate information, and organize communities. The story examines the development of social media campaigns, illuminating how hashtags, challenges, and viral movements have brought awareness of breast cancer to the forefront of digital conversations and fostered a sense of connectivity among people from all over the world.

The tale dives into programs aimed at dispelling myths, encouraging early detection, and cultivating a culture of health, and the significance of educational campaigns takes center stage as a result of this development. By focusing their educational efforts in certain areas, advocates hope to demystify breast cancer, provide consumers with information regarding risk factors and screenings, and encourage individuals to take an active role in their own healthcare. This section emphasizes that raising awareness is not a one-time event but rather a continuous conversation that demands sustained efforts and engagement on the part of everyone involved.

The intersectionality of breast cancer advocacy is also investigated in this chapter.

This is done in recognition of the reality that the impact of breast cancer can be influenced by a variety of characteristics, including gender, race, socioeconomic status, and geographical location. Advocates seek to ensure that awareness and support are inclusive by addressing the particular issues that are encountered by diverse populations. By understanding these intersections, advocates can better address these challenges.

The story comes to a close with a call to action, which acknowledges that advocacy and awareness campaigns are not inactive activities but rather active movements that demand consistent support. The transformative power of advocacy comes in the collective voices that demand change, challenge stigmas, and envisage a future in which breast cancer is not merely treated but also avoidable. This power may be found at both the local and global levels.

Each voice is a note in the symphony of breast cancer advocacy and awareness campaigns, and each campaign is a resonant chord in the overall structure of the symphony. This chapter is an ode to those individuals who have spoken out against injustice, initiated social movements, and paved the road for positive change. It encourages readers to join the chorus, recognizing that through increasing awareness, challenging norms, and campaigning for improved healthcare, we contribute to a future in which breast cancer is not only battled but also vanquished. It does this by inviting readers to join the chorus.

CONCLUSION

A Concluding Statement That Sings a Collective Symphony of Hope and Progress in the Fight Against Breast Cancer

The symphony of breast cancer research is coming to a close, and as we draw the final notes, the resonating theme is one of optimism, perseverance, and communal progress. This narrative weaves together a tapestry that transcends individual experiences and embraces a global community that is united against breast cancer. Beginning with the intricate nuances of understanding breast cancer and moving on to the transformative power of survivor stories, proactive measures in prevention, and amplified voices of advocacy and awareness campaigns, this narrative brings to life a breast cancer fight that spans the globe.

The progression through the chapters demonstrates that breast cancer is more than just a problem related to health; rather, it is the result of a complex interaction involving science, humanity, and collective action. By gaining a grasp of the complexity of breast cancer, we give ourselves the power of information. We also recognize that awareness is not a passive act, but rather a catalyst for early identification, educated choices, and, ultimately, improved outcomes.

The experiences of cancer survivors shine a light on the power of the human spirit to persevere in the face of adversity, bearing witness to the fact that it is possible to weather the storm of a diagnosis and subsequent treatment and emerge on the other side with a sense of renewed fortitude, optimism, and significance. These stories go beyond the confines of the hospital setting and demonstrate that being a cancer survivor is about more than just eliminating cancer cells; it's also about reclaiming one's life, discovering the beauty in the journey, and becoming champions for change.

Recognizing that the journey through breast cancer is not completed in solitude, the chapter that focuses on providing support to loved ones underscores the enormous impact of empathy and connection. The emotional terrain can be navigated with compassion, generosity, and steadfast support from one's family and friends, who become pillars of strength during this time. They can demonstrate that love and connection are essential aspects of the recovery process by collectively redefining what it means to be a part of a community.

The fight against breast cancer has given rise to a call to action, pushing individuals to take an active role in determining their own health destinies by adopting a proactive posture. Lifestyle choices, genetic counseling, early detection practices, and the strength of community participation are all intertwined in a story that emphasizes that prevention is not a far-off ideal but rather a concrete journey, woven into the fabric of daily decisions and societal norms. This narrative emphasizes that cancer prevention is not a faraway ideal but rather a journey that emphasizes the power of community engagement.

The idea that bringing attention to breast cancer is not a solitary pursuit is consistently echoed in advocacy and awareness campaigns, regardless of whether they are local or international in scope. It is a communal symphony where voices join together in harmony, challenging stereotypes, reforming policies, and cultivating a culture in which breast cancer is met with understanding, support, and proactive healthcare measures.

As we come to the end of our investigation, we are brought back to the reality that the battle against breast cancer is a continuing one that is both fluid and rife with opportunities for advancement. Each chapter is like a note in a larger song about hope, a song that is still developing, still resonating, and still inspiring change. We contribute to a future where breast cancer is not simply treated but prevented, where survivor stories become the norm, and where the symphony of hope echoes for generations to come by increasing our awareness of the disease, empathizing with those affected by it, working to prevent it, and advocating for it.

This conclusion should serve as a call to action in the larger fight against breast cancer; specifically, it should be seen as a call to maintain efforts to raise awareness, build support, and advocate for positive change. while they say, "There is strength in unity," and while we negotiate the difficulties of breast cancer, we do so with the common vision of a future where triumph, resilience, and optimism define the breast cancer journey. This gives us the strength to do what we do.